YOUR PELVIC FLOOR

EDUCATION & WISDOM FROM
PELVIC HEALTH PROFESSIONALS
ACROSS THE GLOBE

the
*Inside
Story*

KIM VOPNI — THE FITNESS DOULA

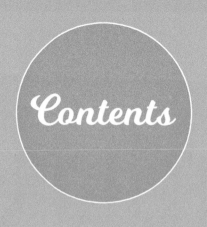

Contents

PELVIC FLOOR WELLNESS IS THE NEW BLACK

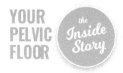

YOUR PELVIC FLOOR

*Y*our pelvic floor is a group of muscles *(3 layers)* that run from the pubic bone *(it is actually a joint called the pubic symphysis)* to the tailbone, as well as the sitz bones. The pelvic floor is a highly vascular *(a large blood supply)*, as well as a highly innervated *(a lot of nerves)*, part of the body. The nerves, muscles and connective tissue work to keep you continent, to provide support to the internal organs *(the bladder, the uterus and the rectum)*, to stabilize the spine and pelvis, and to contribute to your sexual satisfaction. It also plays a major role in childbirth.

Because it is not visible, the pelvic floor is rarely thought of until there is a problem and then it becomes the only thing you think about because it plays such a central role in so much of what you do. Problems will often show up during pregnancy or after childbirth - problems such as incontinence, pelvic pain, organ prolapse, sexual challenges, back pain and/or hip pain. These problems, also known as **pelvic floor dysfunction**, can develop from a variety of reasons such as overuse *(muscles that don't relax and that are tight and weak as a result)*, from under-use *(muscles that lack tone and are weak)*, from injury *(perineal injury or nerve injury from birth, sports, accidents, surgeries)*, or from poor posture and alignment. The pelvic floor is the foundation of your core and deserves a lot more attention than it gets!

Pelvic floor challenges can result from overuse or underuse of the muscles. Here are some of the more common types of pelvic floor dysfunction and tips on how to prevent them or treat them.

Incontinence

A common side effect of pregnancy and birth, *(notice that I said common and not normal)* is **incontinence** – the involuntary loss of urine.

There are a few different types of incontinence. **Stress incontinence** occurs if you are exerting a force like running, laughing, coughing, sneezing, or jumping and urine leaks out a little bit at a time. **Urge incontinence** is when you feel like you have to go all the time, or feel like you can't hold it, and you can't make it to the bathroom in time. **Mixed incontinence** is a combination of stress and urge incontinence.

Incontinence may be a result of weakening muscles, overused muscles or poor timing of the pelvic floor muscles. Risk factors include: being female, obesity, menopause, pregnancy and childbirth, having given birth to more than one child, birth injuries and interventions *(forceps, tearing, episiotomy)*, surgery, chronic coughing, medication, smoking and chronic straining during bowel movements. 50% of women at some point in their life will experience urinary incontinence and 33% will develop regular problems. 3.3 million Canadians suffer from incontinence and only 1 in 12 people seek out treatment because they are embarrassed to talk about it, or don't know that help is available.

Pelvic Organ Prolapse

Pelvic Organ Prolapse is another challenge that is even less known and talked about than incontinence.

50% of women who have had children will have some degree of prolapse and most are unaware due to the few symptoms with this condition in the early stages. Also, 50% of women who have diastasis recti will have some element of pelvic floor dysfunction *(mainly incontinence and prolapse)*.

Of note here is that prolapse does not only occur in women who have had children. Pregnancy and birth increase the risk but it can happen in women who have never been pregnant or had children pointing to other influences such as posture, lifestyle, age, hormones etc. As noted earlier, one of the functions of the pelvic floor is to help keep the pelvic organs in place. The position of the bladder, the uterus and the rectum is partially dependent on the strength and position of the pelvis and pelvic floor muscles. A weakened pelvic floor loses its ability to provide support which

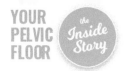
can interfere with the ability to hold the organs in their anatomical position. Unsupported organs will therefore start to descend into and, in severe cases, out of the vagina which is obviously something you want to avoid.

There are four stages of prolapse: early stage prolapse, grade 1 and 2, is often asymptomatic which is why preventive pelvic floor physiotherapy is such a key part of your health care team. When caught at grade 1 or 2, prolapse can be well managed and may even be reversed. **Grade 3** occurs once the organ is at the introitus *(the entrance to the vagina)* and **grade 4** is once the organ is bulging out of the vagina. Once the organ*(s) (you can have more than one organ prolapsing)* get down close to the opening of the vagina or out of the vagina there is no reversing that. Once it's out, it typically becomes a surgical need. This is life altering. Not life threatening but very life altering. Many young women living with prolapse will say "My body is broken." And "Why didn't anyone tell me this could happen?"

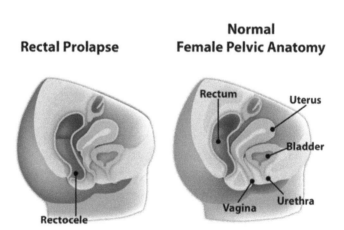

Rectal Prolapse

Rectocele

Normal Female Pelvic Anatomy

Rectum
Uterus
Bladder
Vagina
Urethra

Cystocele Prolapse

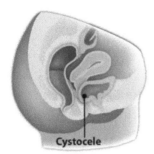

Normal Female Pelvic Anatomy

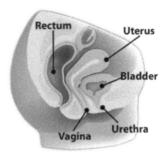

Uterine Prolapse

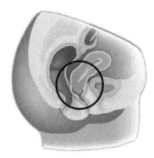

Normal Female Pelvic Anatomy

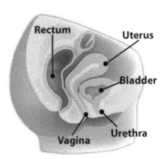

Vaginal Vault Prolapse

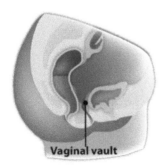

Normal Female Pelvic Anatomy
(post-hysterectomy)

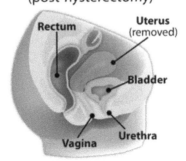

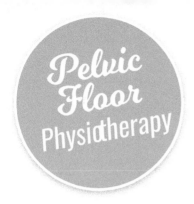

Pelvic Floor Physiotherapy

— the most unknown and underused women's health tool

Pelvic Health Physiotherapy is 80% effective for treating urinary incontinence and research shows that physiotherapy involving internal assessment and treatment should be the first line of defence for urge and stress incontinence. Pelvic Floor Physiotherapists *(also known as pelvic health or women's health physiotherapists)* have taken specialized training in internal evaluation and treatment. They can design a program that is individualized to your needs, which may include addressing pelvic floor muscle weakness, tightness or both.

They start by taking a detailed history about your symptoms, fluid intake, any previous pregnancies/surgeries/injuries and other medical conditions. They then provide education on where your pelvic floor muscles are located and how your posture directly affects the activation of these muscles. An external exam is then conducted, which looks at your core stability including whether an abdominal separation *(diastasis)* is present. Research has shown that over half of the women with incontinence also have an abdominal separation. The next step is an internal pelvic exam involving observation, and palpation *(feeling)* of the soft tissue and muscles outside and inside the vagina and rectum. The physiotherapist will assess the pelvic floor muscles for tension, tone, strength, power and endurance, as well as the presence of any trigger points in the muscles.

PELVIC FLOOR PHYSIO

JST DO IT.

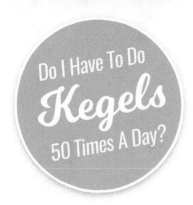

Do I Have To Do *Kegels* 50 Times A Day?

In some cases, **Kegels** may be the training method of choice but 30-50% of women are doing kegels *(pelvic floor muscle training)* incorrectly. Kegels were developed by **Dr. Arnold Kegel** and were well intentioned, however they are not always the answer to incontinence, even when performed correctly. Pelvic floor muscles can be tight *(just like any other muscle in our body)*, or restricted *(from scarring)* or have trigger points *(causing pain)*.

Women with tightness, pain or restrictions will not benefit from Kegels. The other thing to note about kegels is that they are typically done while sitting in a car or late at night in bed – usually rushed and in poor posture. Kegels will never be effective like this. Incorporating pelvic floor exercise *(contractions and relaxation)* into movement is the best way to train your pelvic floor.

The only way to know if your pelvic floor is tight or weak or both, is to have an internal assessment conducted by a trained Pelvic Health Physiotherapist who can guide you through an exercise program that shows you how to do a kegel properly, and also how to incorporate pelvic muscle exercise into movement.

Kegels are cool

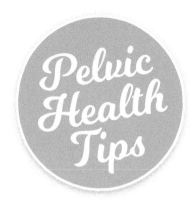

- Avoid constipation. Repeated straining is similar to mini childbirth for your pelvic floor, which can cause these muscles to become weak over time. Check out squattypotty.com.

- Drink water consistently throughout the day. Restricting fluids can cause your urine to become concentrated, which can irritate your bladder and signal you to empty more often than you should

- Avoid bladder irritants like artificial sweeteners, acidic foods, chocolate, alcohol, caffeine.

- You should urinate between 5-9 times a day. Don't *'pee just in case'*; Learn to wait until your bladder is full before going to the bathroom.

- Learn 'The Knack'. Tighten your pelvic floor muscles before you cough, sneeze or lift heavy items.

- See a pelvic health physiotherapist at least once a year.

- Avoid exercises that make you leak until your function has been restored and then gradually return to that activity.

- Pay attention to your cycle. Estrogen levels change throughout your monthly cycle. Right before, during, and right after your period is generally when your estrogen levels are at their lowest, making you more likely to experience leakage during that time in your cycle.

- Talk to your daughters, sisters, aunts, friends — all women need to know this information!

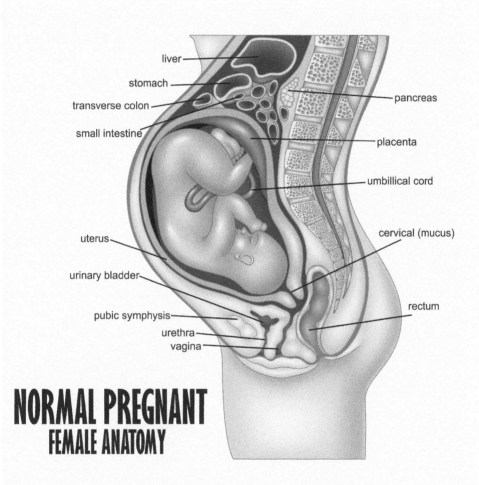

liver

stomach

transverse colon

small intestine

pancreas

placenta

umbillical cord

uterus

cervical (mucus)

urinary bladder

pubic symphysis

urethra

vagina

rectum

NORMAL PREGNANT
FEMALE ANATOMY

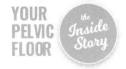

YOUR
PELVIC
FLOOR

the
Inside
Story

YOUR PELVIC FLOOR IN PREGNANCY

*T*he abdominal wall, pelvic floor, and low back undergo increasing strain with the weight of the growing baby, the expanding uterus, and the additional fluids. Adding to this strain is the effect of the hormones on ligament laxity, making the joints less stable. All these changes contribute to alterations in your posture that can affect your alignment, and therefore the function of your core and surrounding muscles. The pelvis will often start to tip anteriorly, the shoulders round as the breasts grow, and the head juts forward. Actually this forward head, rounded shoulders posture is the one most people live in all day, every day, without even being pregnant! Truth be told, many women actually start their pregnancy with elements of core dysfunction. *Huh— who knew?!*

FRONTAL SECTION OF PELVIS

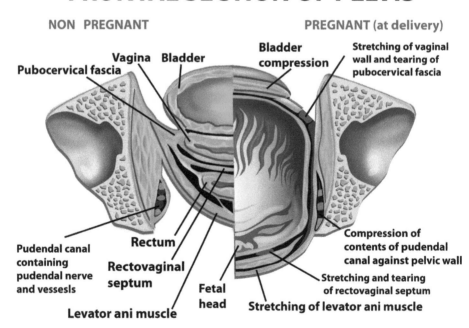

NON PREGNANT

PREGNANT (at delivery)

Pubocervical fascia
Vagina   Bladder

Bladder compression
Stretching of vaginal wall and tearing of pubocervical fascia

Pudendal canal containing pudendal nerve and vessesls

Rectum

Rectovaginal septum

Levator ani muscle

Fetal head

Compression of contents of pudendal canal against pelvic wall

Stretching and tearing of rectovaginal septum

Stretching of levator ani muscle

In pregnancy, the centre of gravity is shifting. Women try to counteract this forward shift in body weight by leaning back, pushing the hips forward, and clenching the butt muscles. The tailbone tucks and the hips thrust forward, and stability is then attempted by gripping in the butt and the obliques. These are non-optimal strategies, and are the body's way of trying to stabilize itself when the muscles that should be supporting the core are not working properly because of poor posture and alignment.

They are compensations, and they need to be prevented or changed. These poor core stability strategies alter the breathing and overuse the posterior pelvic floor and move the pelvic floor into a less supported position. They also inhibit and weaken the glutes and increase intra-abdominal pressure, which is not good for the abdomen or the pelvic floor. Add to this the extra weight from the growing uterus and you have a pelvic floor that is overworked and out of position! The good news is that even if you go into pregnancy with an element of core dysfunction, and even if you already have some aches and pains, you can take steps now to reverse them and prevent these things from becoming a bigger problem.

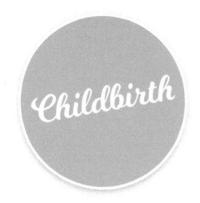

Childbirth, whether vaginal or surgical, can greatly affect the core. Vaginal birth causes extensive strain on the pelvic floor muscles, connective tissue, and nerves. It alters the pelvic landscape which can affect the overall feel and function of the pelvic floor. Even in the absence of tearing or an episiotomy, dysfunction can occur due to the excessive pressure, stretch, and compression that takes place during the first and second stages of labour. Many women also face other interventions that increase the potential of tearing and episiotomy—interventions such as forceps, vacuum extraction, and prolonged pushing in the second stage of labour. The act of pushing can also stress the abdominal wall and if diastasis recti has not already occurred in pregnancy, it may occur during the pushing phase of labour.

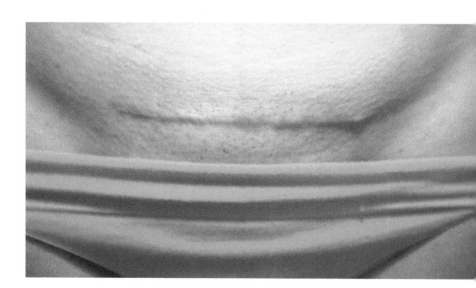

A **surgical birth, or cesarean section,** involves incisions into the abdominal wall and the uterus which alters everything—the ligaments, the organs, the muscles, the tissues. A cesarean birth, while it may offer a small protective affect with regards to pelvic organ prolapse *(more on that later)* changes the body and often leaves the postpartum body with bigger challenges.

Birth is a **very physical event** that needs to be prepared for and recovered from. Unfortunately women are using very intense activity during pregnancy to get 'fit for birth' and then using equally intense activity to 'get their bodies back'. All of this is at the detriment of their pelvic floors and abdomens. To prepare for the marathon of birth, 'sport specific' training should be used – low impact, endurance based, strength and release work will best prepare the body for the task at hand. Close attention needs to be paid to the recovery. Little to no upright movement in the first week is ideal coupled with abdominal wrapping and warm nurturing foods. The weeks following should involve slow purposeful restorative core work with gentle walking. At **6 weeks postpartum** EVERY new mom should see a pelvic floor physiotherapist to retrain the core followed by a gradual progression back to regular activities between 6 and 12 months. Encouraging young women to be proactive, to prepare, recover and restore will mean future generations will maintain optimal pelvic floor health for life.

Birth Wisdom

BIRTH IS LIKE A MARATHON and just like you need to train for a marathon, you need to train for birth. Cardio, release work, and strength and endurance training are all essential, and special attention needs to be paid to the pelvic floor and abdomen.

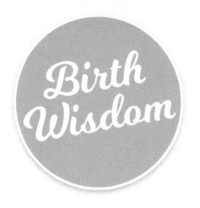

– KIM VOPNI
PORT MOODY,
BC CANADA
WWW.PELVIENNEWELLNESS.COM

AVOID LABORING ON YOUR BACK OR SEMI-SEATED.

Be upright, move, change positions... even with an epidural! And for best results: give birth on hands and knees, rocking back toward a heel sit with contractions to push... yes, even with an epidural!

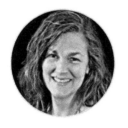

– SUSAN STEFFES, PT
AUSTIN TEXAS, USA
WWW.SUSANSTEFFESDPT.VPWEB.COM/

see a pelvic physiotherapist

DURING PREGNANCY *(or even earlier during pre conception)* **TO CHECK HOW YOUR PELVIC FLOOR IS FUNCTIONING WHICH WILL HELP WITH A SMOOTHER PREGNANCY, LABOUR/DELIVERY AND POSTPARTUM RECOVERY.**

– ANITA LAMBERT, PT
PETERBOROUGH,
ON CANADA
WWW.HOLISTICHEALTHPHYSIO.COM

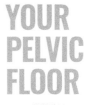

YOUR PELVIC FLOOR

the Inside Story

EDUCATION & WISDOM
FROM PELVIC HEALTH
PROFESSIONALS
ACROSS THE GLOBE

"

Studies show it may take years or even decades for some problems such as incontinence and chronic pain to show up after childbirth.

Once postpartum, always postpartum.

"

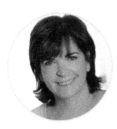

— MARIANNE RYAN, PT

NEW YORK, NY USA
WWW.BABYBODBOOK.COM

• •

"

HERE'S THE DEAL. YOU'RE NOT MADE OF STEEL. GET REAL NEW MOM, AND HEAL YOUR SEAL!

New Moms often think that just because they are given the green light to exercise 6 weeks after birthing a baby (or babies), they are somehow completely ready to go back to doing exercises they were doing before they got pregnant. Your pelvic floor and the rest of your core needs time to heal and start working properly again after the many changes that occurred with pregnancy and childbirth.

It may feel like a bore, when you think you're ready for more, but please, I implore, if you've had one babe or four, explore the right way and strengthen your pelvic floor!

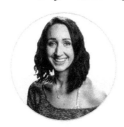

"

— JEN OLIVER

WINDSOR, ON CANADA
WWW.LOVEFITMAMA.COM

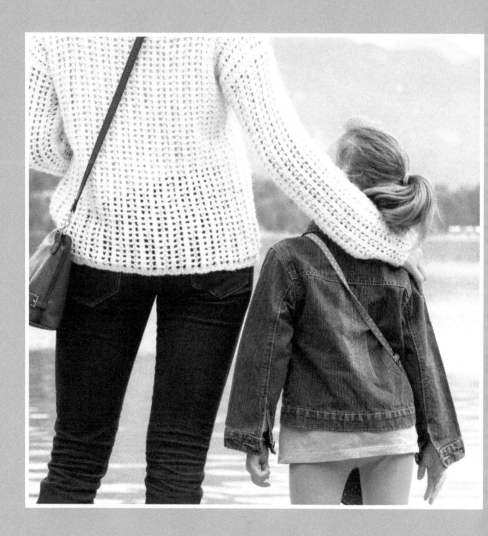

YOUR PELVIC FLOOR IN MOTHERHOOD

Following pregnancy and childbirth, the pelvic floor landscape has changed. Even if there were no interventions, no tearing or surgery, the pelvic floor and overall core is different. Initially women may ignore signs of pelvic floor dysfunction because they think it is *'normal'* after having kids, because they are embarrassed or simply because they don't know that help exists.

Scar tissue, muscle imbalance, organs out of position, leaking, back pain, knee pain, hip pain — these are all common postpartum pelvic floor challenges that can be helped! Pelvic floor physiotherapy is an essential first step and can be life changing. You will learn things about your body that you won't believe you have not known before.

Motherhood is busy and demanding, and many women are so focussed on caring for their family that they forget to care for themselves. They ignore signs and symptoms, they stop having sex, they avoid certain activities and are soon feeling depressed, isolated and alone not knowing that it is their pelvic floor that has contributed to the way they feel.

The pelvic floor plays a role in pelvic and spinal stability, incontinence, in sex — these are all really important aspects of our life and it is not until there is a problem that women realize the importance of their pelvic floor. It is typically not even thought about until there is a problem... and then it is the only thing a woman can think about.

Prevention is ideal, but it is never too late to optimize your pelvic health and improve the way it works, which means you can get back in the sack, you can participate in the activities you want and you do not have to plan your day around toilets.

Prioritize YOU and your pelvic health. See your pelvic floor physiotherapist annually to keep it in check and mother with confidence!

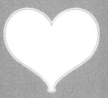

KEEP
CALM
AND
KEGEL
ON

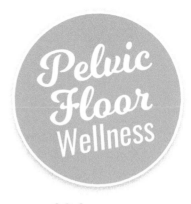

Pelvic Floor Wellness

The action of a pelvic floor contraction is *close and lift*. Most anatomical diagrams show everything sitting up with the organs lined up like soldiers, when in reality the orientation of you pelvic floor and organs is forwards. If you stand up and feel where your hip bone is you will feel that your pelvis is tilted forwards and if you put a finger on your anus think about where it will 'lift' to – towards your pubic bone.

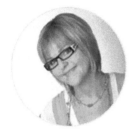

— FIONA ROGERS, PT

SIPPY DOWNS, QUEENSLAND AUSTRALIA
WWW.PELVICFLOOREXERCISE.COM.AU

Pelvic Floor Wellness: We need to start talking about pelvic health and wellness. Let's put aside all our pre-conceptions, insecurities and discuss all the topics openly, without judgement so that we can live long healthy lives without pelvic dysfunction.

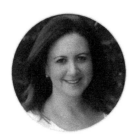

— NELLY FAGHANI, PT

NEWMARKET, ON CANADA
WWW.PELVICHEALTHSOLUTIONS.CA

WWW.PELVIENNEWELLNESS.COM

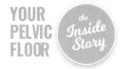
"

As a physical therapist and yoga therapist, it has been extremely valuable to combine physical therapy and yoga when addressing a variety of pelvic health issues. I have found that focused meditations such as 'body scanning' and 'pelvic diaphragmatic breath awareness' have been instrumental in creating a higher awareness of the pelvic floor, which is the first step prior to releasing, engaging or controlling the pelvic floor muscles (PFM's).

One of the best pelvic health tips I recommend to men and women is to practice what I call the "Toilet Meditation". There are a few specific parts to the meditation; but in summary, it is simply being completely present and aware when performing your toilet duties! As you sit, scan the entire body and notice any areas of tension or physical sensations. Try to stay present in your body and aware of your breath, observing any thoughts that take you away from the present moment.

Focus on observing the natural rhythm of both the respiratory and the pelvic diaphragms as you breathe, releasing the PFM's and taking your time. We often rush when we urinate, and may not always fully empty our bladders. This can potentially result in a cascade of unwanted issues, or exacerbate existing issues such as persistent pelvic pain dysfunctions, over active bladder or incontinence, to name a few.

Part of optimal pelvic floor health starts with awareness, breathing, and ability to release the PFM's. *The "Toilet Meditation" is an easy way to start incorporating healthy pelvic floor habits* without adding another item on your 'list of things to do' during your day!

"

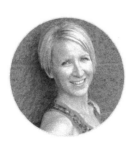

— SHELLY PROSKO, PT
SYLVAN LAKE, AB CANADA
WWW.PHYSIOYOGA.CA

"

During attempted vaginal penetration, if it feels as if
your partner is "hitting a wall", whether it be difficulty inserting
a penis, dildo, finger, or sex toy, stop! Pelvic floor disorders
can make vaginal penetration difficult or impossible, and
persevering through the pain will worsen the situation.

"

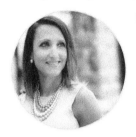

— DR. LORI BROTTO

VANCOUVER, BC CANADA
WWW.BROTTOLAB.COM

"

*I wish everyone knew that they should not go
to the bathroom "just in case."*
This typically leads to increased urinary urge and frequency
during the day AND can also cause one to have to wake up in the
middle of the night to go. I give my patients a challenge - try to
avoid going to the bathroom just in case. Rather wait at least
2-4 hours and within 2 weeks, there should be a change noticed.
This can require baby steps at first, but it can be life changing.

"

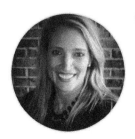

— TRACY SHER, PT

ORLANDO, FL USA
WWW.SHERPELVIC.COM
WWW.PELVICGURU.COM

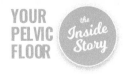

*Be consistent with your exercises
and soon it will become routine
like brushing your teeth.*

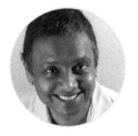

— GOWRI ATKINSON, PT
COQUITLAM, BC CANADA
WWW.ACTIVELIVINGPHYSIOCLINIC.CA

Once you have found your floor and coordinated it with the breath,
it is time to talk work. ALL WORK IS NOT EQUAL.
THE ACTIVITY YOU ARE DOING DICTATES THE WORK
YOUR FLOOR HAS TO DO i.e.: putting on your socks does not require
the same pelvic floor (PF) activation that moving a fridge does.
Once your PF is automated, or at least something you don't have to think of
as often, you can ramp up the work when needed
(moving the fridge) and hopefully breathe and move with ease
and trusting your PF is firing just as much as it needs to.

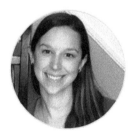

— LAURA APPS, PT
AJAX, ON CANADA
WWW.WOMENSHEALTHPHYSIO.CA

Never blow your nose when sitting on a toilet peeing. Blowing your nose contracts the PFM and your floor should be relaxed to let the pee out.

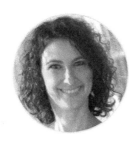

— JULIA DI PAOLO, PT

TORONTO, ON CANADA
WWW.BELLIESINC.COM

One of the earliest signs of vulvar or vaginal cancer can be skin changes. Most women are aware of the benefits of doing regular SBE's (self breast exams) but few (unfortunately) are doing regular vulvar self exams.

Position yourself comfortably, propped up in bed. Make sure your hands are clean Don't use any creams or lotions, as this may interfere with your ability to detect any changes. Holding a mirror in one hand and use your other hand to separate the labia and look at your vulva. Check the clitoris and the surrounding area.

Then move down to the vaginal opening. Check the small folds of skin to the left and right. Now move down to the area around the anal opening because vulvar disease can spread to here. If you notice:

- Any lumps, bumps or skin changes
- Itching
- Pain
- Burning sensation, especially after urinating
- Any unusual discharge
- That you bleed after sex
- That you bleed between periods OR after menopause

Then make an appointment to see your doctor.

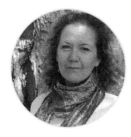

— MICHELLE LYONS, PT

FORE, WESTMEATH, IRELAND
WWW.CELEBRATEMULIEBRITY.COM

WWW.PELVIENNEWELLNESS.COM

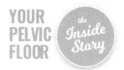

YOUR
PELVIC
FLOOR

the
Inside
Story

"

If we were animals walking on all fours, prolapse wouldn't be an issue because our organs would have great support from the pubic bone and muscular wall of the abdomen. But since we walk upright, we have the effect of gravity weighing down on our organs which rely on strong pelvic floors to support them from beneath. There are little things you can do throughout the day to improve their support.

Sitting and standing in an upright posture with your pelvis tilted forward and buttocks lifted slightly helps keep the organs nicely supported by the pubic bone rather than being positioned over the vaginal opening. Over the long haul, this can make a big difference to how much downwards pull gravity has on your organs.

"

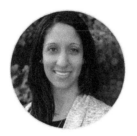

— MUNIRA HUDANI, PT

TORONTO, ON CANADA

WWW.BOSNARHEALTH.COM/?PAGE_ID=300

"

There's no shame in finding out you are incontinent, the shame comes when you don't do anything about it but before buying products and gadgets, blind off the net, get and see a women's health physio for proper advice and help first. Your pelvic floor needs proper training, BEST TO SEEK TRAINING FROM THE PROFESSIONALS i.e. women's health physio's, *they know what they are doing and teach you how to best train yourself.*

"

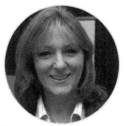

— GAYNOR MORGAN

SOUTH WALES, UK

WWW.INCOSTRESS.COM

Learning to use your core correctly is not just for while you're 'doing your exercises'. Those few minutes of focus each day are great for re-connecting with your body and your muscles, but *the time when you really need to look after your core, is the everyday stuff, when you have a child, heavy bags or the laundry to pick up!*

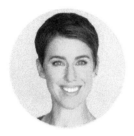

— WENDY POWELL
CORNWALL, UK
WWW.MUTUSYSTEM.COM

Work to get your ribcage stacked on top of your pelvis in standing. Too often we stand with our hips pressed too far forward. This causes our hips, quads and abdominal muscles to work too hard and alters the position of our pelvic organs relative to one another which can contribute to hip, back and pelvic dysfunction, pelvic organ prolapse, incontinence, and many other pain and function issues.

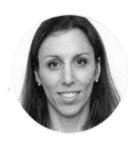

— TRISH GIPSON, PT
VANCOUVER, BC CANADA
WWW.ENVISIONPHYSIO.COM

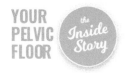

"

The pelvic floor muscle is my favorite muscle in the body! Take a moment and appreciate what a typical day in the life of this muscle might entail.

All day long this amazing muscle is silently working to protect us and we are usually oblivious to its critical contributions. Day and night it must contract and relax immediately, properly and efficiently to react to every pressure change in our body, from subtle to large. This could be as little as during a hiccup or when standing up from sitting, to protecting us when we need to lift something heavy or keeping us safe during a 10 km run. The pelvic floor muscle works all day long to support us in healthy biomechanical postures and seamlessly transferring forces through the pelvis from our legs and trunk every time we move. This muscle is always 'on the job' ensuring we don't accidentally pee or pass gas when we laugh or sneeze and ensuring we have a good and complete void and bowel movement when we decide the time is right. This muscle assists our diaphragm in respiration so it is literally working with every breath we take!

And then, after working all day long, this wonderful muscle gives us the fulfilling orgasm we deserve to complete a perfect day.

Hmmm... what a muscle! Isn't it worth it to make sure you keep your pelvic floor muscle happy and healthy?

See a qualified pelvic floor physiotherapist for a customized pelvic floor exercise program that's best for your pelvic floor muscle and enjoy the benefits.

"

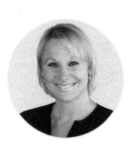

— DR. KELLY BERZUK
WINNIPEG, MB CANADA
WWW.NOVA-PHYSIO.COM

"

The pelvic floor and core have a role in:

STABILITY - BALANCE - DIGESTION - ORGAN SUPPORT - RESPIRATION - MOBILITY
ELIMINATION - REPRODUCTION - EMOTION

Typically, we think pelvic floor/ core issues are present when we see symptoms like incontinence, pelvic organ prolapse, low sex drive or poor sexual response or pain in the pelvis. However, we also know that the following less known symptoms are also indicative of poor pelvic/core function;

- *Poor balance or physical performance*
- *Irritable bowel, poor digestion, constipation*
- *Pain in back, hips, shoulders, the jaw*
- *Poor posture or misalignment, fatigue*
- *Mood disorders*

If unaddressed, any one of these problems can lead to other wider psychological issues such as social isolation, relationship and intimacy issues, poor self esteem and a decrease physical activity.

We need to understand that our pelvic floor and our core are complicated and require so much more than kegels! To broaden our perspective - the pelvic floor, respiratory diaphragm, deep abdominals and the back muscles act like instruments in an orchestra. They all need to do their part and play together to create beautiful and safe movement music. Of course we can't forget about the conductor of this orchestra, the brain! The brain coordinates this complex movement music through many feedback loops involving such things as hormones, nutrition, the nerves, emotions, somatic receptors and more. We are so much more than muscles and bones. The key is to create an environment of availability within each of our bodies to allow the all of the systems to work together.

See a Certified Pelvic Health Physiotherapist **to learn about how you can play beautiful music within your body and orchestrate beautiful movement!**

"

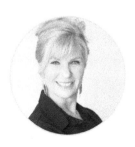

— CHERYL LEIA, PT
NORTH VANCOUVER, BC CANADA
WWW.PHYSIOTIQUES.COM

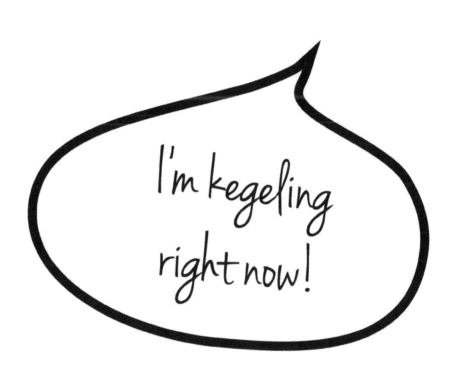

Cardio

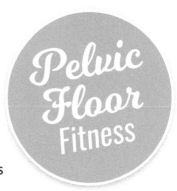

Swimming, cycling and walking are all great choices if you are living with pelvic organ prolapse. Gentle, low/no impact activities will prevent additional strain on the ligaments and muscles that support the internal organs. Pay attention to your posture while you cycle – opt for padded cycling shorts and a gel seat so you can sit with your pelvis as close to neutral as possible. When walking, try to incorporate some hills if possible and avoid the treadmill if you can as it doesn't mimic our natural gait. You may also want to consider transitioning to minimalist shoes where your foot is as close to barefoot as possible. Positive heeled shoes *(when the heel is higher than the forefoot)* shift your pelvic alignment and can cause mal-alignment of the organs as well.

Body Weight Exercise

To get a good workout, you don't need equipment – all you need is your body. Some of my favourite body weight movements are **bridges, donkey kicks, and wall push-ups.** Bridges work the glutes and hamstrings while inverted so it removes the strain on the pelvic floor. Donkey kicks work the glutes and hamstrings as well, with the elbows down, it is also an inversion of sorts. Wall push-ups put the body in a forward lean with downward pressure. Be sure to add the **Core Breath** to these moves – ready exhale to pre-contract the pelvic floor and then press up or away. See the **Core Breath Video** at http://www.pelviennewellness.com/pages/videos

Weight Training

If you love to lift weights, it is advised to reduce the weight to avoid the additional strain on the pelvic floor. Choose lighter weights and up the reps. Supine and side lying positions can help reduce the effect of gravity on the pelvic floor. Try crook lying tricep extensions to work the backs of your arms. For your shoulders, lean

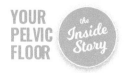

on a ball and do lateral raises. For your biceps get on your knees leaning over a ball and do preacher curls. Whenever you are weight training you should pre-contract your pelvic floor before you lift or exert a force. Add in core breathing to every move.

Hypopressives™

The term **'HYPOpressive™'** refers to a decrease or reduction in pressure. This form of exercise, now being referred to as **low pressure fitness™**, reduces pressure to the thoracic, abdominal and pelvic cavities, where traditional abdominal exercises, gravity, as well as the majority of our daily activities are **HYPERpressive** — they increase intra-abdominal pressure. We need some intra-abdominal pressure to help stabilize our spine. Sometimes we lose the ability to manage these pressures and this is what can then lead to dysfunctions of the pelvic floor.

Hypopressives™ are a specific set of poses that create a decrease in pressure and amplify the hypopressive effects, lift the internal organs and improve posture. In the pose, an apnea *(a temporary cessation of breathing)* and a false inhale are added after a full exhale to create a vacuum affect resulting in a decrease of pressure within the thoracic, abdominal and pelvic cavities.

http://www.pelviennewellness.com/pages/hypopresive-method

Stretching and Release Work

Ensure your daily regimen *(even on rest days)* include hamstring stretches and calf stretches. By lengthening the muscles in the back of the legs, it will allow the pelvis to maintain its neutral position. Sitting all day and wearing heels can shorten the backside and contribute to core dysfunction. Leg up on the wall pose is a great pose that eliminates gravity and opens up the pelvis and hips. Supine butterfly is another favourite of mine to help open up the hips.

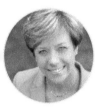

Imagine your pelvic floor like a twisted door, how well would it open and close? It is important to remove the twists within and between the thorax and pelvis for optimal function of the pelvic floor.

— DIANE LEE, PT

WHITEROCK, BC CANADA

WWW.DIANELEE.CA

UNTUCK YOUR BUTT FOR BETTER FLOOR FUNCTION:

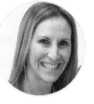

The position of your pelvis effects how you contract your PFM and TA. In a sway back position commonly seen in females, the PF muscle can't function at optimal. Keep your pelvis in neutral – that's with a slight anterior tilt, so think a little 'Donald Duck' but not too much. Think about this during the day and whilst exercising.

— LORRAINE SCAPENS

AUCKLAND, NEW ZEALAND

WWW.PREGNANCYEXERCISE.CO.NZ

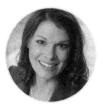

When doing pelvic floor exercises, make sure that once you have 'got' the connection to the muscles, you start integrating them into core exercises and functional activity. It is not useful if the only time you can activate the muscles is flat on your back. I say that the pelvic floor is part of a "neighbourhood" of muscles and to be successful at pelvic floor strengthening, you need to integrate these muscles back into the neighbourhood so that they can be used functionally. :)

— KATHLEEN
SHORTT, PT

TORONTO, ON CANADA

WWW.INBALANCEPHYSIO.CA

WWW.PELVIENNEWELLNESS.COM

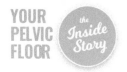

"

The best way to avoid pelvic floor dysfunction is to maintain a good posture and deep squatting is a great way to do this. Build up your squatting tolerance over time, making sure you maintain a straight back and belly breathe throughout.

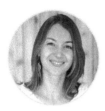

— ANNIKEN CHADWICK, PT

VANCOUVER, BC CANADA
WWW.ANNIKENCHADWICK.COM

"

Choose a fitness style that blesses and benefits your pelvic floor. If your workout is wrecking your pelvic floor and not restoring, it's time to step back and reassess your program and goals. Definition isn't worth dysfunction. If your exercise regimen is increasing your incontinence issues or widening your diastasis recti, then it's too much for your body in your present state, and it's time to seek one-on-one rehab with a specialist and switch to restorative exercises. And this frustrating time when you need to slow down to move ahead again? Yeah, it's just a season, friend. Trust that if you give your body what it needs right now, it will give you what you need later. Honor your body's limits today, and your body will honor you by expanding those limits tomorrow. This isn't forever. You will get stronger again. But right now you need to put yourself back together with gentle movements and wholesome foods. And I believe you will look back on restful seasons in your life with fondness once you learn to embrace them.

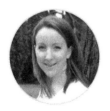

— BETHANY LEARN

VANCOUVER, WA USA
WWW.FIT2B.US

"

Work on ribcage mobility to ensure proper breath & pelvic floor health.

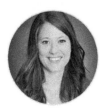

— ANDREA PLITZ, PT

OTTAWA, ON CANADA
WWW.ANDREAPLITZPT.COM

Remember that "working out" your pelvic floor can be as simple as breathing. The pelvic diaphragm works with the respiratory diaphragm. On an inhale, the pelvic diaphragm releases and on an exhale it returns to it's normal position. Repeat as many times as you breathe. Awareness can win half the battle.

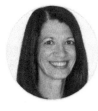

— CAROLYNE
ANTHONY
SOUTH ORANGE, NJ USA
WWW.THECENTERFORWOMENSFITNESS.COM

When you lift weights, "lift" your pelvic floor first. Adding additional weight load (especially heavy) can create a lot of intra-abdominal pressure as well as downward pressure on to your pelvic floor in an effort to get enough power to lift. This can be dangerous if you don't recruit your pelvic floor properly and create a strong foundation. *Get assessed by a pelvic floor physiotherapist especially if hitting the weight room.*

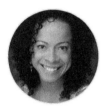

— SAMANTHA
MONTPETIT-HUYNH
TORONTO, ON CANADA
WWW.BELLIESINC.COM

EXPAND YOUR MOVEMENT DIET:

A common saying is variety is the spice of life and I truly believe this is the case in our fitness. *To spice up your exercise routine, I dare you to try something new* - bend yourself into a pretzel at yoga, plie with poise and grace at ballet, find some head space by taking a long walk in the fresh air or challenge your strength and stamina in a weights session.

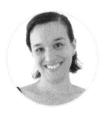

— JENNI
VAN DEN BERG
BRISBANE, AUSTRALIA
WWW.ZIPRFIT.COM.AU

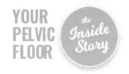

If you are practicing kegels it is important to begin by fully relaxing the muscles of the pelvic floor, and the hips, the glutes and the belly. Make sure to practice this relaxation in between each kegel repetition. This will improve your awareness of contraction and relaxation of the pelvic floor muscles.

Stand with your legs hip distance apart and softly bend one knee while keeping the foot planted; let the hip and pelvis follow the movement. Extend the knee and try the same movement on the other side. This gentle biomechanical movement can help address low back pain and issues of tension in the pelvic floor.

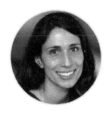

— FRANCESCA AMBROCICHUK, PT

HALIFAX, NS CANADA
WWW.SYNERGYPHYSIOPILATES.COM

Paddle board season! Engage and lift the pelvic floor as you push the oar through the water. You'll feel an increase in core power.

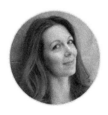

— DUSTIENNE MILLER, PT

BOSTON, MA USA
WWW.FLOURISHPHYSICALTHERAPY.COM

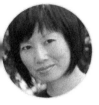

Remember no pain or leakage is 'normal' and should be assessed – the earlier the better! It continues to amaze me how well pain clients respond to pelvic floor physiotherapy. It works amazing and having pain free sex keeps women and their partners very happy (and smiling) – *as does running free with no leaks!*

— YOLANDA TSANG, PT

OTTAWA, ON CANADA
WWW.YOLATESREHAB.COM

10 MINUTES PER DAY:

Don't view exercise as a chore or a form of punishment. Instead think of it as a life habit, much like brushing your teeth or personal hygiene. We exercise because we love ourselves, our bodies and our health, and so we can be our best. Start by setting aside 10 minutes daily for some kind of pelvic floor exercise. Once you have mastered making that a habit, I am sure you will end up adding time without even realizing, just because it makes you feel good!

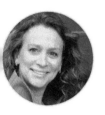

— ELISABETH PARSONS

UXBRIDGE, ON CANADA
WWW.FIT4YOU.CA

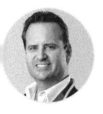

Bladder control is a fitness issue.

— DR. BRUCE CRAWFORD

RENO, NV USA
WWW.PFILATES.COM

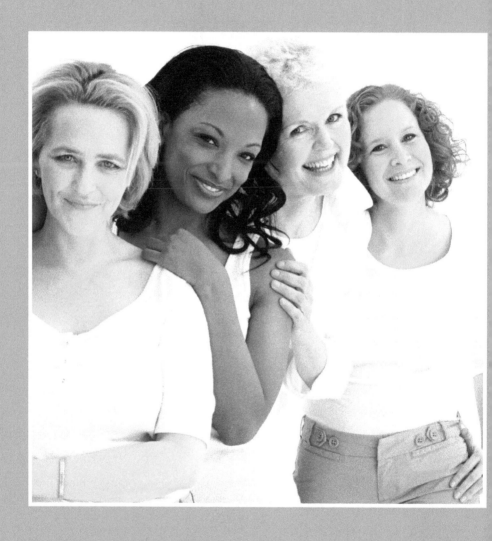

YOUR PELVIC FLOOR IN MENOPAUSE

*T*he pelvic floor undergoes more changes as you approach and enter menopause. You are older *(and wiser)*, there have been more posture changes, perhaps surgeries or accidents, and now there is also the influence of **hormones**.

As you age, your bladder becomes less elastic and does not stretch like it used to. So as the bladder fills with urine, this loss of stretch can irritate the bladder muscle causing you to feel like you need to go all the time. Combined with weaker pelvic floor muscles, this can present some challenges.

The loss of the hormone estrogen can contribute to vaginal dryness as the lining of the vagina produces less mucus. Estrogen also helps your pelvic floor to be strong, supple and stretchy, which gives you greater control over your bladder and bowel function. Estrogen depletion can contribute to more urgency, frequency of urination and sometimes urge urinary incontinence. During menopause, your estrogen levels naturally decline, which can lead to increased incontinence. Additionally, during the time leading up to menopause, called "premenopause" or "perimenopause", your estrogen levels begin to gradually decline.

Many women find they begin to gain weight with the onset of menopause and because the pelvic floor muscles support most of your body weight, as you gain it, your pelvic floor needs to carry it.

Many women have had a **hysterectomy** and this can cause incontinence for a couple reasons:

1. Removing the uterus changes the pelvic landscape and can cause the muscles to weaken and sag, which can cause incontinence;

2. Your ovaries are responsible for creating most of the estrogen in your body. If the ovaries are removed during a hysterectomy, this can lead to a significant drop in estrogen levels.

WWW.PELVIENNEWELLNESS.COM

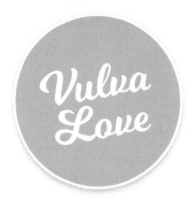

Vulva Love

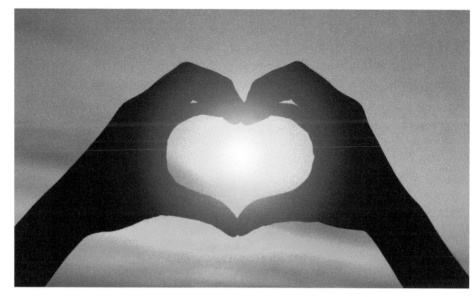

"

After 18 years of working as a Pelvic Health Physiotherapist, it amazes me how little we know about taking care of our vulvas. So many of our daily habits can contribute to unnecessary discomfort – itchiness, burning and even pain with intercourse. There are still so many social stigmas and misconceptions surrounding our vulvas. My wish would be that we teach proper vulvar skin health to our young girls before they start their menses! Let's start these good habits at a young age.

So what do you need to know? First, have a look down there! Get to know your vulva. Every vulva and folds of labias are unique and beautiful just like a snowflake.

DEVELOP SOME GOOD VULVAR SKIN HABITS:

- AVOID USING SOAP ON YOUR VULVA. *This is so drying to your skin. When our estrogen levels lower, such as before our menses, during breastfeeding and after menopause, the skin of the vulva becomes more sensitive and dry. Try not to scrub. All you need is water to wash your vulva. Please be gentle. The vulva does not need a vigorous scrub down!*

- WEAR COTTON UNDERWEAR *to allow the skin to breathe.*

- AVOID WEARING UNDERWEAR AT NIGHT.

- MINIMISE INFECTIONS BY WIPING FROM FRONT TO BACK *after you void or having a bowel movement.*

- STAY AWAY FROM ANY VAGINAL DOUCHING PRODUCTS! *The vagina is self-cleaning and does not need to be cleaned!*

- *If you have sensitive skin,* USE MENSTRUAL PADS THAT ARE COTTON BASED *or organic during your menses.*

- AVOID USING MENSTRUAL PADS IF YOU SUFFER LOSS OF BLADDER CONTROL. *These pads wick away a lot of moisture from the skin of the vulva and should only be used during menstrual cycles.*

- USE A GOOD LUBRICANT WITH INTERCOURSE, *especially if you have any discomfort with intercourse. Avoid those that use parabens and glycogen since these are irritating to the vulva.*

- MOISTURIZE! *This helps seal in moisture or adds moisture to the skin. Use a natural moisturizer, like coconut oil and apply some to the skin of the vulva.*

So please be kind to yourself and take good care of your vulva, inside and out!

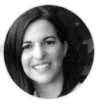

—MARIE-JOSÉE
FORGET, PT

NORTH BAY, ON CANADA
WWW.GATEWAYPHYSIO.COM

YOUR
PELVIC
FLOOR
the
Inside
Story

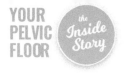

Every vulva is unique and beautiful.

Take a mirror and look at your vulva to be able
to monitor change. Love your vulva!

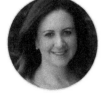

— **NELLY FAGHANI, PT**
NEWMARKET, ON CANADA
WWW.PELVICHEALTHSOLUTIONS.CA

There are at least 11 muscles in the pelvic floor network! The
important actions of the pelvic floor are to hug in, pull up, push
out, open and close.

*In addition to supporting all of the internal organs, your
pelvic floor muscles are key actors in the play of sexual
arousal and function.* Beyond core health, mastering the
movements of the pelvic floor can increase your turn on and
support you in learning to have a variety of orgasmic releases.

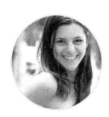

— **LARA CATONE**
VENICE, CA USA
WWW.LARACATONE.COM

It is just as important to moisturize
your vagina as it is your face.

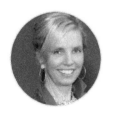

— **MAUREEN
MCGRATH**
VANCOUVER, BC CANADA
WWW.BACKTOTHEBEDROOM.CA

"

While we live in a busy world and rushing seems to be a daily sport, please resist the temptation to force or push pee out. When doing so, you can bulge your pelvic floor outwards which does not help to maintain good muscle tone. Instead sit down, relax your sphincter and let gravity do its thing. You may not save time but you could reduce your pelvic floor stress.

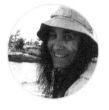

— TRISH BRUNELLE,
BHSC, PT

BARRIE, ON CANADA
WWW.GETMOVINGPHYSIO.COM

"

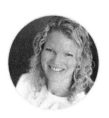

Don't go pee just in case.

— DR. SINEAD DUFOUR

MILTON, ON CANADA
WWW.THEWOMB.CA

"

Observe your perineal area (with a mirror) every few months or so.

Not only can you spot something that looks out of the ordinary, you can also gain valuable perspective and connection with your vulva: IT IS NOT A FORBIDDEN ZONE! Men get to see their parts up front and centre. We just have to go a little out of our way to look at ours. And while you are down there smile and do a kegel... it might just wink back ;)

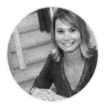

— GAYLE HULME, PT

CALGARY, AB CANADA
WWW.LAKEVIEWPHYSIO.CA

I

♥

My pelvic

FLOOR

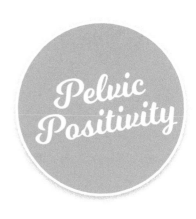

Pelvic Positivity

> If you always do what you've always done,
> you'll always be what you've always been!
> *Dare to improve yourself!*

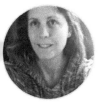

— KAILI BAAS, PT

NORTH BAY, ON CANADA
BAASPHYSIO@GMAIL.COM

Women around the world suffer in silence with symptoms they don't understand. Stigma has veiled pelvic organ prolapse (POP) in silence for nearly 4000 years, but as women navigating this extremely common condition come together to talk out loud about the impact to their quality of life, we will lift the veil, establish POP awareness, and generate the next big shift in women's health directives.

Pelvic organ prolapse is without a doubt the biggest secret in women's health. We have so much more to do; we have so much more to learn. Women with POP are hungry for hope. We move forward side by side.

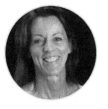

— SHERRIE PALM

FOUNDER/EXECUTIVE DIRECTOR
ASSOCIATION FOR PELVIC ORGAN PROLAPSE SUPPORT

MUKWONAGO, WI USA
WWW.PELVICORGANPROLAPSESUPPORT.ORG
WWW.SHERRIEPALM.COM

WWW.PELVIENNEWELLNESS.COM

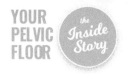

YOUR PELVIC FLOOR — the Inside Story

"

Remember. You were YOU before you were a mom. Taking care of yourself, reconnecting with yourself — mind, body and spirit, is a way of being able to give your BEST self to your family. Pelvic floor health is so much more than just kegels. *It is about giving you the confidence to live the life that you want to live to the fullest!*

"

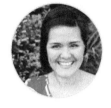

— KAREN SAN ANDRES, PT
OAKVILLE, ON CANADA
WWW.ELLEPHYSIO.COM

"

If someone out there is suffering with any type of pelvic pain, genital pain, pain with sexual activity and related conditions, *there's so much HOPE to getting better.* I promise. The trickiest and most frustrating part is that many health professionals are not trained in these types of conditions. So, my best advise is to continue to seek out specialists who really understand how to treat this and don't give up. Most patients see 8-10 healthcare professionals before getting help from someone like me. *I'm on a mission to make sure more people know there is hope and more clinicians are trained to provide the best care.*

"

— TRACY SHER, PT
ORLANDO, FL USA
WWW.SHERPELVIC.COM
WWW.PELVICGURU.COM

WWW.PELVIENNEWELLNESS.COM

Copyright © 2016

BLUEBERRIES & JELLYFISH

#kegelcues

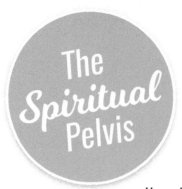

The Spiritual Pelvis

There is so much more to the pelvic floor than the physical aspects. The pelvis is an area women carry most of our emotional pain.

Unresolved emotions like grief, loss, guilt, shame, blame, anger and/or resentment from past or present trauma can be held as dense energy in the pelvic area. This dense energy becomes a block interfering with energetic flow and blood circulation. *If we don't heal our emotional blocks, the physical body will never heal fully.*

Through my intuitive readings I look at our 5 bodies. The physical body is the most obvious one. We also have the emotional, mental, spiritual and energy bodies. They all feed into and influence each other and often disease, illness or physical pain is rooted strongly in one, but will influence the others. If you don't get to the root of the disharmony, then everything becomes a temporary fix or a band-aid. For example clients with back pain often have an emotional root that is influencing the physical body. For example, if one doesn't feel supported by their spouse, it often shows up as a lack of support by their body. If they feel unstable in their life, their spine is often unstable. It is important that we focus our attention and intention on healing the physical, mental, emotional, energetic and spiritual aspects in order to return to a state of harmony and vibrant health.

The first key is awareness. If you feel that you have unresolved emotional or energetic blocks in your body, I recommend you find an intuitive healer, energy worker, reiki practitioner or someone who can help you heal and re-align your mind, body and spirit. Trust your intuition. It will lead you on your path to healing and wholeness. *Follow the directions of your heart, one bread crumb at a time.*

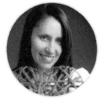

— SUE DUMAIS
LANGLEY, BC CANADA
WWW.HEARTLEDLIVING.COM

Over the years working as a physio, I've learned that sometimes the most obvious thing is the most overlooked. We often jump right into treating one thing or another, but in the words of that famous song from that famous musical, "let's start at the very beginning". And what is the very beginning?

Awareness.

I'm talking about the ability of you and I to tune in, feel, perceive, and sense — to sense where we are in space, to feel the subtleties of our daily postures and positions, to appreciate the nuances in our movements, and to notice the connections between seemingly unrelated body parts.

Awareness is the starting point in pelvic health physiotherapy because it is essential to everything that we subsequently do. Developing that sense of mind-body awareness means that you can really know, reconnect to, and hopefully appreciate the amazing system that is your body. It allows you to take control over your pain or dysfunction, instead of letting it control you. It means that you can begin to make changes and improvements to your health on the micro and macro levels. It ultimately helps to rewire and retrain your brain, neural pathways, and motor patterns. When you begin to develop this perceptual ability, it really is amazing how much more you can feel and the overall impact on your pelvic health. Feeling is the key to healing.

So before starting anything else, before breathing, or visualizations, or kegels, or any other exercise, I usually say something that goes a little bit like this: "*Close your eyes, quiet your mind, concentrate, and feel...*"

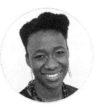

— IBUKUN AFOLABI, PT

LONDON, ON CANADA
WWW.THEMAMASPHYSIO.COM

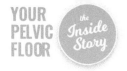

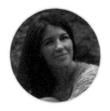

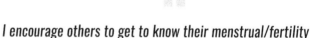

Pelvic health affects not only the body, but also the mind and spirit. **Seeking emotional support for pelvic health symptoms that can impact so many aspects of a woman's life is essential for optimizing wellness.**

— **KEIRA BROWN**
TORONTO, ON CANADA
WWW.SACRALHEALING.COM

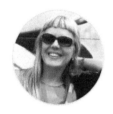

I encourage others to get to know their menstrual/fertility cycles, and not just to see them as being about periods. *There is an entire universe of helpful and fascinating insights available to us when we chart our cycles,* **especially if you take the time to cross-reference what you learn with a lunar calendar. Our bodies are amazing, beautiful, life-giving mysteries: let's see them as a resource to be cherished, not a problem to be solved.**

— **MADELEINE SHAW**
VANCOUVER, BC CANADA
WWW.LUNAPADS.COM

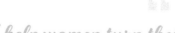

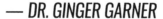

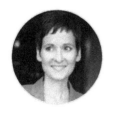

I help women turn their grief into courage **— to find their authentic voice and strength, through the lens of integrated yogic care in physical therapy**

— **DR. GINGER GARNER**
EMERALD ISLE, NC USA
WWW.GINGERGARNER.COM

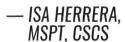

Your path to healing lies within you.

You have to be strong and have courage in the face of adversity. Listen to the messages from your body, have a strong intention to awaken the healer within you. Always remember you are more than just the story of your pain, and that true healing must occur on all aspects your being, emotional, physical, and spiritual.

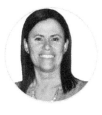

— ISA HERRERA,
MSPT, CSCS

NEW YORK, NY USA

WWW.RENEWPT.COM

On any journey, there are bound to be obstacles that we need to navigate. Remember to stay focused on your destination, ask for directions and keep moving. With an open mind, the detours we take can be as rewarding as the path we had first set out for ourselves. **My journey led me to the** Hypopressive® **technique, a form of training I use and teach to put the power back in the hands of women diagnosed with pelvic floor dysfunction such as prolapse.**

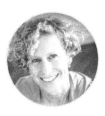

— TRISTA ZINN

PERSONAL TRAINER

TORONTO, ON CANADA

WWW.HYPOPPRESSIVESCANADA.COM

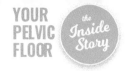

I **leave you with 2 requests.** It is my sincere hope that you will take at least one tip from this book and put it into action *(the one I hope you choose is to see a pelvic floor physiotherapist... just sayin').* My second request is that you pass this book on to all the women in your life because like you, they deserve to know.

Yours in pelvic health,

Kim

For more information visit
www.pelviennewellness.com.

Pelvienne Wellness, Inc. offers products
and services to women for pelvic health in
pregnancy, motherhood and menopause.

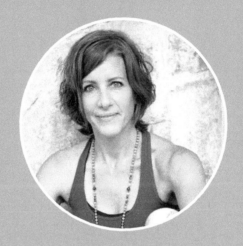

Kim Vopni is a mom, an entrepreneur and a passionate preacher of pelvic health! She is the owner of **Pelvienne Wellness Inc.** and co-founder of **Bellies Inc.** With a strong desire to empower and educate women about proactive and restorative health, Kim uses many platforms to deliver her message including public speaking, her popular event **Kegels and Cocktails™**, writing articles and through social media. You can find her online on **Facebook, Twitter & Instagram.**

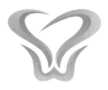

CPSIA information can be obtained
at www.ICGtesting.com
Printed in the USA
LVHW070250250919
632039LV00004B/22/P